100 Plus

Simple Homemade

Organic Body Scrub

Recipes

For Face And Body Exfoliating

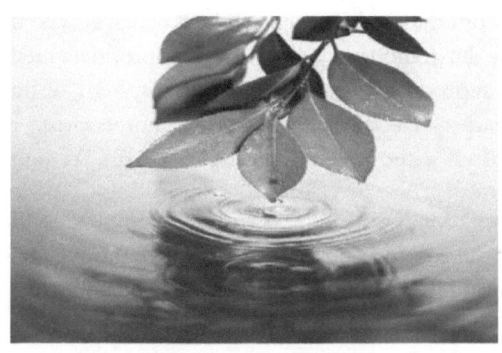

SANDY COMFORT

ISBN-13:978-1508971696

ISBN-10:1508971692

DEDICATION

To the famous five: Kim, Dora, Sue, Mirry and of course my humble self,
Thank you for the wonderful times we had exfoliating our skin.

TABLE OF CONTENTS

INTRODUCTION

I love my skin. That is because it is soft and so smooth. The secret is that I exfoliate regularly.

Our skin is a living organ. It breathes and lives and requires a lot of care much more than any other organ in the body. Let's not forget the role it also plays in protecting us from the elements.

Exfoliating is the primary treatment for your skin. It is simply the process of getting rid of the dead skin cells that are on the skin's surface and when these dead skin cells are taken off, the healthier and younger looking skin resurfaces.

If you want to have a radiant and smooth skin, exfoliating is a must. Failure to exfoliate leaves your skin covered with dead cells that muck up the surface and gives you a dull and older look. When you repeatedly ignore this process, foundation applied won't smooth over your skin cleanly. Moisturizers won't soak in properly either. Exfoliating should be a vital part of our day to day beauty routine.

Facial scrub is important for breaking white -heads, cleansing the skin and dislodging build-up in the pores. It smoothens and refines the texture of the skin. It enhances blood flow to the body as well.

How Often Should You Exfoliate?

Most health professionals say that two times a week is sufficient. For people with sensitive skin, less is required. Do not scrub too hard and too often if you have a sensitive skin otherwise you will end up removing healthy cells and your skin will look red and feel sore. Simply rub the particles firmly but gently in circular motions. Too much exfoliation will irritate the skin.

Women with oily skin need to exfoliate more frequently than women with dry skin. However, if your skin becomes irritated or dry after exfoliation, you shouldn't scrub so hard. Simply reduce how often you exfoliate. It might just be that you are allergic to the products you used.

Use exfoliating cleansers that contain sugar, sea salt, walnuts, ground almonds, seeds or other grainy components.

Exfoliating The Entire Body

While it is good to exfoliate the face, the entire body needs to receive similar treatment. This is because the skin sheds up to 50,000 dead cells per minute. Not all dead cells fall off; some of them simply build up to clog pores or leave you with a rough skin.

Exfoliate your arms, neck, back, chest and back to prevent body acne. When you exfoliate, the dead skin cells that are in the parts of the body where you've waxed or shaved will be prevented from plugging up follicles. It can even out skin tone and keeps your skin soft and hydrated.

Procedure

• Wet your body in the shower from head to toe.

• Start with the soles of your feet and work your way up your body.

• Remove rough spots and calluses on your feet using a pumice stone. If you have very rough feet, add a cup of milt to a basin of warm water, stir and soak your feet inside it for 30 minutes before entering the shower.

• Apply your scrub to your gloves or loofah. Scrub your body in a circular motion beginning with the bottoms and work your way up. Don't scrub too hard when you get to the bikini area because of the sensitive nature of the skin.

• Use a body brush to scrub your back and those places that cannot easily be reached.

• Scrub your face gently. Pay attention to your mouth and eyes but you must use an exfoliating product meant for the face because it is gently that those made for the body.

• Remember your hands; they should look and feel soft too.

• Rinse your body using lukewarm water.

• Step out of the shower.

• Pat your face dry with a clean towel after exfoliating.

• Apply a moisturizing lotion all over your body

Ensure you use facial moisturizers and body lotions that contain alpha or beta hydroxy acids because they help in removing dead skin cells.

Tips:

After exfoliating, apply sunscreen if you are going out in the sun. You do not want the fresh skin to be damaged by the sun especially since it may be slightly irritated.

Preserve the smoothness and avoid breakouts by using a non comedogenic moisturizer.

Don't scrub your face too hard, this can cause damage to and hurt your skin.

Do not exfoliate if you have an open wound or cut or if you are sunburned.

Although a variety of body scrubs are available on the market these days. They are filled with addictives and preservatives that could harm your skin in the long run. It is advisable to be cautious of what we absorb into our skin. It is unrealistic to eat organic foods and then introduce chemicals into our bodies through our skin. The solution to a wonderful skin is in your kitchen, not the store!

The Double Boiler Method

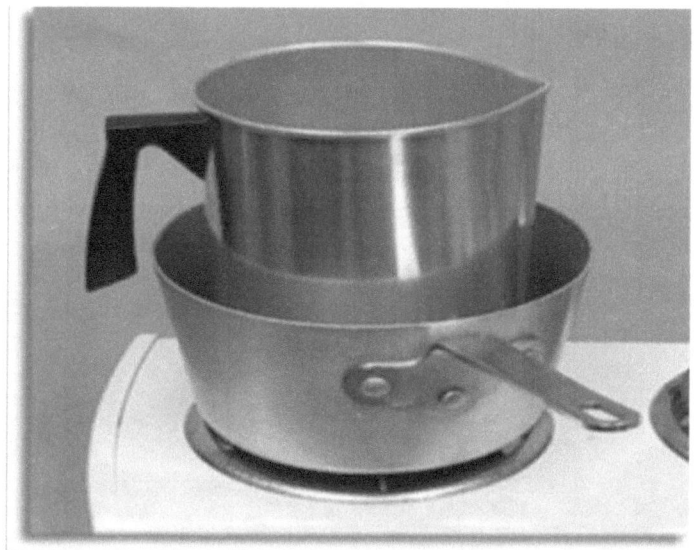

Some of the recipes in this book require the use of the double boiler method to make.

A double boiler method is effective for heating materials gently without scorching or burning them. You may either buy one but they are quite simply to make on your own.

• Get two pots, the smaller one should fit into the big one.

• Fill the big pot with some water.

• Place a one inch high sheet metal ring into the big pot. This will help the small pot to sit perfectly.

• Place the small pot on top of the big pot of water. It should not touch the water.

• As the water boils, the heat will be transferred to the smaller pot which has been filled with whatever you want to melt or cook.

• This can either be done in the oven or on the stove

The recipes in this book are great and incredibly amazing. You will even be tempted to eat them!

I have used organic ingredients and created recipes that you will definitely love. They are tested and proven. It is my belief that you will enjoy using them as much as I have.

Essential Oils

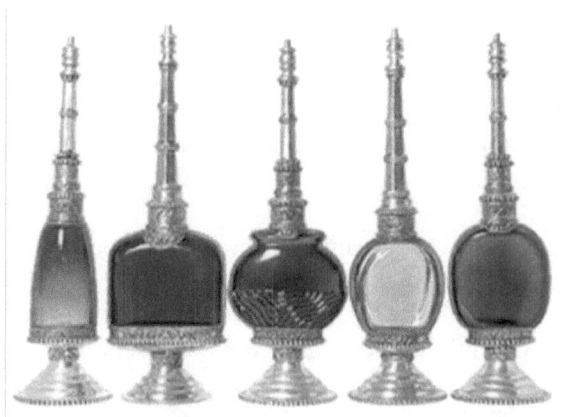

Essential oils are aromatic oils popularly used in the cosmetic industry. They are highly concentrated and have rejuvenating and healing abilities — the best treatment for your skin. These oils are extracted from the leaves, flowers, stem, seeds and roots of plants, the bark of trees as well as the peel of citrus fruits. They do not dissolve in Aloe Vera juice or water but dissolve only a little in vinegar.

If wrongly used, essential oils are harmful and this is the reason they must be kept out of children's reach. They are flammable as well and should never be placed near fires.

Essential oil should be stored in a dry and cool place. This enables it to retain its potency for 5 to 10 years. The citrus oil are an exception, however, because it only retains its healing properties for 6 to 12 months.

Be familiar with the properties and contraindications of every essential oil before using it.

Safety tips to remember when preparing your own body scrubs:

• Undiluted essential oils must never be directly applied to the skin.

• They should not be taken internally because they are highly concentrated and toxic if ingested.

• Some essential oils may cause allergic reactions and skin irritation.

• Some essential oils are not suitable for pregnant women and individuals with health conditions like asthma and epilepsy.

• Essential oils like citrus oils and bergamot may cause skin sensitivity to sunlight, even when diluted. They should not be applied on sunny or extremely hot days.

• If the oil accidentally gets into your nose or eyes while working with it, flush out the affected part immediately using unscented fatty oil like olive, soybean, almond or peanut.

• To determine possible allergic reactions of a particular oil, carry out a skin patch test. Mix one or two drops of the essential oil and ½ to 1 teaspoon of base oil in a small bowl. Dab a small portion in the inside of your elbow, behind your ear, inside your upper arm, or behind your knee. Cover it for 24 hours with a band aid. If no irritation occurs, then the oil is safe to use.

Below are a few essential oils that are widely used in cosmetics. You can be creative and add to the under-listed to create your own unique blend.

Lemon and Bergamot should not be used on sensitive skin

Lasmine, Chamomile, Rose and Geranium should not be used during pregnancy

Eucalyptus, Frankincense, Lavender, Neroli, Palmarosa, Petitgrain, Orange, Rosewood, Sandalwood, Ylang Ylang

Base Oils

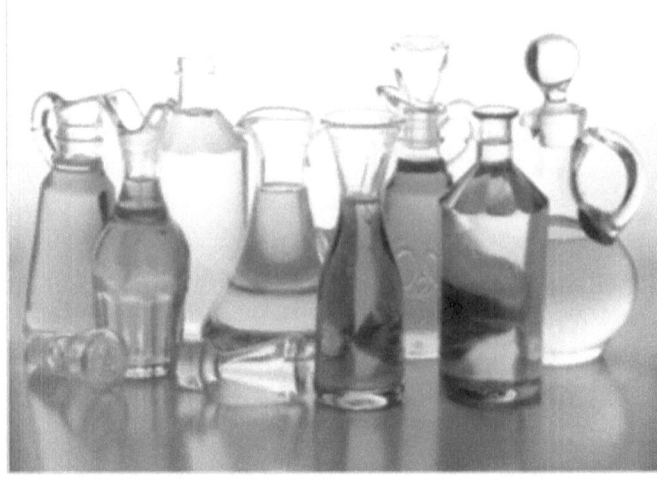

Base oils (also known as carrier oils) are primarily used in diluting essential oils before applying them to the skin. They are derived from fruits, vegetables, beans, seeds and nuts. They are generally cold-pressed vegetable oils without their own scent and this is why they can serve as perfect counterparts for essential oils.

Grapeseed, Jojoba, Sunflower, Sweet Almond, Avocado Peanut, Sesame and Apricot kernel are examples of a few of them.

Organically grown base oils which have been extracted naturally and processed minimally are the best for personal care recipes. These particular oils have not been exposed to very high temperatures, bleaching, deodorizing or chemical extraction procedures that can alter or destroy antioxidant properties, natural aromas, flavors and beneficial vitamins.

Check the labels for keywords like cold-pressed, expeller pressed or refined before you buy.

Remember to always check the expiry date on the bottle and return immediately if the oil is bad. Ensure you make your purchase from reliable retailers that have a high inventory turnover.

Skin professionals sometimes use the terms slide and slip to describe the way oil product glides onto the skin. It indicates that the oil is neither rapidly absorbed nor sticky. This is the kind of base oil that is just right to use as a face or body massage oil. Soybeans oils and organic almond have thinner texture and are therefore excellent massage base oils. Jojoba oil also serves as balancing body oil.

Unlike essential oils, carrier oils have a short shelf life and becomes rancid once opened.

Fragrance Oils

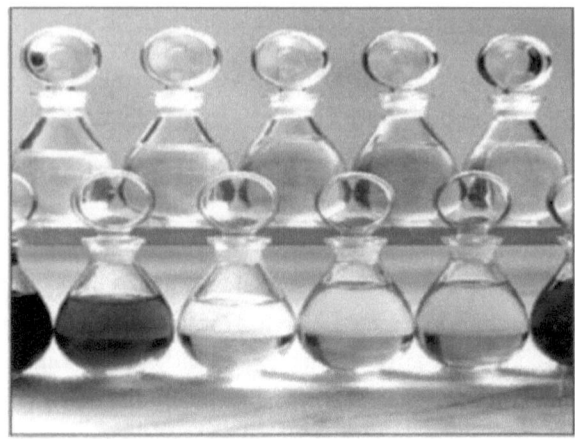

Fragrance oils, also called aroma oils, flavor oils or aromatic oils are natural essential oils that have been diluted with a carrier like mineral oil, vegetable oil or propylene glycol.

Fragrance oils are used to add a variety of scent to those fruits that do not produce essential oil such as mango, strawberry and watermelon. It is possible to even make one that will smell like chocolate! They serve as a fantastic fragrant addition to body scrubs and lotions.

However, before using these aromatics, be sure to read and follow the instructions provided on the label. And like essential oils, only a few drops are required to produce wonderful fragrant results.

Butters – Shea, Cocoa, Mango

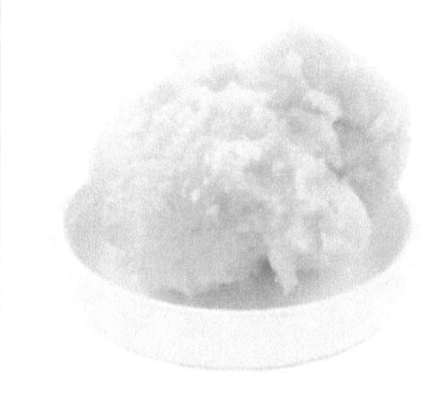

Shea nut butter is ivory-colored. It is a natural fat extraction from the fruit of the Shea tree. This fruit is called a nut and has an avocado-like seed in it. It is from this seed that Shea butter is extracted. Its uses are diverse.

• It has soothing and moisturizing effects.

• It prevents certain sun allergies.

• It protects the skin from harmful UV rays.

• It helps capillary circulation and cell regeneration.

Cocoa Butter is an aromatic solid butter from the seeds of the cacao tree which is extracted and roasted. This solid butter softens at body temperature. It adds a thick, rich and creamy consistency to body scrubs, lotions, creams and soaps which improves the skin's elasticity by helping to reduce dryness.

Mango Butter is cold pressed and rendered from the mango tree's seed kernel. It works effectively as a mild lubricant for the skin and has beneficial moisturizing properties. It is an excellent quality base ingredient perfect for body care products. It is also loaded with essential fatty acids.

SUGAR BODY SCRUBS

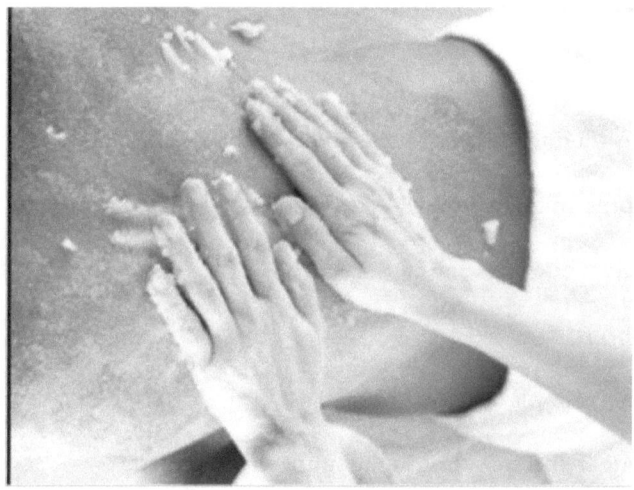

Sugar scrubs are highly recommended for individuals who have sensitive skin. They are gentler than salt and remove dead skin cells, dirt and toxin leaving the skin with a healthy and revitalized glow.

Sugar has anti-aging properties because it produces an alpha hydroxy acid known as glycolic acid which has been proven by generations to rejuvenate skin. Sugar scrubs give your skin a natural appearance and a younger glow.

Mango Colada

Ingredients:

Coconut oil (1/2 teaspoon)

Coconut fragrance oil (1/4 teaspoon)

Mango fragrance oil (1/4 teaspoon)

Pineapple fragrance oil (1/4 teaspoon)

Organic white sugar (1 cup)

Directions:

Mix oils into plastic bowl or glass

Add sugar and mix thoroughly until well blended.

Shelf Life: Store in a tightly sealed container for about a month.

Orange Sunrise

Ingredients:

Melted cocoa butter (2 tablespoons)

Warmed olive oil (4 tablespoons)

Orange juice (4 tablespoons)

Essential orange oil (2 drops)

Organic brown sugar (1 cup)

Directions:

Blend all the ingredients with a blender until fluffy and light.

Blend again if the mixture separates.

Shelf life: Store in a jar or a tightly-capped bottle. Refrigerate for up to 2 weeks.

Sweet Avocado

Ingredients:

Almond oil (5 drops)

Ripe avocado (1)

Organic white sugar (3/4 cup)

Directions:

Blend almond oil and pour into avocado. Add sugar and use a hand held blender to mix until smooth.

Shelf life: Use immediately.

Jasmine Rose

Ingredients:

Grape- seed oil (10 teaspoon)

Patchouli essential oil (7 drops)

Jasmine essential oil (4 drops)

Rose essential oil (2 drops)

Organic white sugar (1 cup)

Directions:

Combine all the ingredients in a bowl.

Shelf Life: Store for up to 6 months in an air tight container.

Grape Soufflé
Ingredients:

Green grapes (1 cup)

Honey (1 teaspoon)

Egg yolk (1)

Organic white (1 cup)

Directions:

Crush green grapes to pulp. Add egg yolk and honey. Use a hand mixer to whip together

Shelf Life: Store for 24 hours in an air tight container.

Chamomile Petitgrain
Ingredients:

Chamomile essential oil (3 drops)

Petitgrain essential oil (2 drops)

Organic brown sugar (1 cup)

Dried chamomile flowers (1/4 cup)

Directions:

Combine all the ingredients in a bowl.

Shelf Life: Store for up to a month in an air tight container.

Violet Vibrations
Ingredients:

Coconut oil (2 ounces)

Violet fragrant oil (4 drops)

Organic white sugar (1/2 cup)

Red food coloring (optional, 1 drop)

Blue food coloring (optional, 1 drop)

Directions:

Mix ingredients together.

Shelf life: Store for up to a month in an air tight container.

Sugar And Spice
Ingredients:

Baking soda (1/2 cup)

Organic white sugar (2 tablespoons)

Organic ground cinnamon (1 teaspoon)

Organic ground ginger (1/2 teaspoon)

Organic ground cloves (1/4 teaspoon)

Almond oil (2 tablespoons)

Directions:

Combine the dry ingredients in a bowl. Then, add the almond oil. Mix them all together until well blended.

Shelf Life: Store for up to a month in an air tight container.

Apricot Honey Butter
Ingredients:

Kernel oil (10 oz apricot)

Cocoa butter (2 oz)

Organic brown sugar (1 cup)

Organic honey (1 tablespoon)

Directions:

Heat the cocoa butter in the double boiler top until it is melted.

Remove from heat and add the rest of the ingredients.

Beat with a wooden spoon till it is smooth and cooled.

Shelf life: Put in a glass jar, close tightly and refrigerate for 1 month.

Jasmine And Aloe

Ingredients:

Apricot kernel oil (1/4 cup)

Cocoa butter (1 teaspoon)

Coconut oil (1 teaspoon)

Aloe Vera gel (1 teaspoon)

Jasmine fragrance oil (5 drops)

Organic brown sugar (1 cup)

Directions:

Combine ingredients into a bowl and mix thoroughly.

Shelf life: Store in glass jar for up to one month.

Brown Sugar And Almond

Ingredients:

Ground almonds (1 handful)

Brown sugar (2 tablespoons)

Honey (2 tablespoons)

Directions:

Squash almonds in a food processor. Add egg yolk and honey. Use a hand mixer and whip together.

Shelf Life: Store for up to 1 week in an air tight container

Green Tea And Honey

Ingredients:

Honey (2 tablespoons)

Green tea bag (1 organic)

White sugar (1 cup organic)

Almond oil (2 tablespoons)

Directions:

Place sugar in a medium sized mixing bowl. Tear open green tea bag and add to it. Stir to combine.

Next, add the almond oil and mix. Lastly, add 1 tablespoon of honey at a time and mix well.

Shelf life: Refrigerate and use within 1 week.

Spring Fever

Ingredients:

Frankincense essential oil (3 drops)

Lime essential oil (2 drops)

Rose essential oil (2 drops)

Organic white sugar (1 cup)

Directions:

Mix ingredients together in a large bowl.

Shelf Life: Store for up to 6 months in an air tight container.

Sandalwood Rose

Ingredients:

Rose essential oil (2 drops)

Sandalwood essential oil (5 drops)

Ylang Ylang essential oil (2 drops)

Organic brown sugar (1 cup)

Directions:

Combine ingredients in a bowl.

Shelf Life: Store for up to 6 months in an air tight container.

Wheat and Oats

Ingredients:

Organic white sugar (1/2 cup)

Olive oil (2 teaspoons)

Rolled oats (1/4)

Wheat germ (1/4)

Directions:

Mix ingredients together in a large bowl.

Shelf Life: Store for up to 1 month in an air tight container

Grapefruit and Sugar
Ingredients:

Organic brown sugar (1/2 cup)

Sunflower oil (2 teaspoons)

Organic white sugar (1/2)

Vitamin E (1/2 teaspoon)

Grapefruit essential oil (3 drops)

Directions:

Mix ingredients together in a large bowl.

Shelf Life: Store for up to a day in an air tight container.

Herb
Ingredients:

Honey (1/4 cup)

Dry sage (1 teaspoon)

Dry thyme (1 teaspoon)

Dry rosemary (1 teaspoon)

Organic white sugar (1 cup)

Directions:

Combine ingredients and store.

Shelf Life: Store for up to a week in a sterilized glass jar.

Vanilla Almond

Ingredients:

Whole almonds (1/3 cup)

Almond oil (1 tablespoon)

Vanilla fragrance oil (1/8 teaspoon)

Organic white sugar (1 cup)

Directions:

Pour almonds into a food processor or chopper. Then chop till particles are fine.

Combine with the sugar and oils.

Shelf Life: Store in a tightly sealed container. It lasts for up to 2 months

Vanilla Patchouli

Ingredients:

Organic brown sugar (1 cup)

Vanilla fragrance oil (20 drops)

Patchouli essential oil (5 drops)

Ylang-ylang essential oil (5 drops)

Directions:

Mix ingredients together in a large bowl.

Shelf Life: Store for up to 6 months in an air tight container.

Pineapple Passions
Ingredients:

Ripe pineapple (1 cup)

Organic white sugar (1 cup)

Passionflower oil (3 drops)

Sunflower oil (1 tablespoon)

Directions:

Puree cucumber in blender. Then add oils to a mixing bowl of sugar. Mix thoroughly.

Shelf Life: Store for up to 1 week in an air tight container

Cucumber Ylang Ylang
Ingredients:

Ripe cucumber (1)

Organic white sugar (1 cup)

Ylang Ylang essential oil (2 drops)

Sunflower oil (1 tablespoon)

Directions:

Puree cucumber in blender. Next add oils to a mixing bowl of sugar. Mix thoroughly.

Shelf Life: Store for up to a week in an air tight container.

Bergamot Neroli

<u>Ingredients:</u>

Organic white sugar (2 ½ cups)

Almond oil (1/2 cup)

Shea butter (1 tablespoon)

Bergamot essential oil (2 drops)

Neroli essential oil (1 drop)

<u>Directions:</u>

Combine the almond oil and sugar in a large bowl and mix well. Then add the Shea butter and whip/ mix/ with a hand held blender on high speed for about 3minutes. You will have a grainy paste.

Shelf Life: Store in a tightly sealed container for up to 2 months

Strawberry Banana Bliss

<u>Ingredients:</u>

Banana (1 ripe)

Pineapples (1/4 cup)

Strawberries (1/4 cup)

Apricot kernel oil (2 tablespoons)

Organic white sugar (1 cup)

Directions:

Puree fruit in a blender. Mix fruit with sugar and oil.

Shelf Life: Store for up to 3 days in an air tight container

Tea Tree Temptations
Ingredients:

Sunflower oil (8 teaspoons)

Jasmine oil (6 drops)

Tea tree oil (2 drops)

Neroli oil (2 drops)

Organic white sugar (1 cup)

Directions:

Mix ingredients together in a glass jar.

Shelf Life: Store for up to 2 months in an air tight container.

Fresca
Ingredients:

Tangerine fragrance oil (7 drops)

Lemon essential oil (4 drops)

Organic white sugar (1 cup)

Directions:

Combine ingredients in a bowl.

Shelf Life: Store for up to 6 months in an air tight container.

Snow In The Summertime
Ingredients:

Sugar (1/2 cup)

Olive oil (2 teaspoons)

Heavy whipping cream (1/4 cup)

Directions:

Mix ingredients together in a large bowl and use a hand mixer to mix till light.

Shelf Life: Store for up to a day in an air tight container

Maya Papaya
Ingredients:

Papaya (1/2)

Lemon or lime juice (1/2 teaspoon)

Honey (1 teaspoon)

Organic white sugar (1 cup)

Directions:

Puree papaya in a blender. Next, add lemon juice to papaya and blend again. Add the honey and papaya to the sugar in mixing bowl. Mix well

Shelf Life: Store for up to a day in an air tight container.

Cinnamon Celebration
Ingredients:

Organic white sugar (1/2 cup)

Ground cinnamon (1/2 teaspoon)

Almond oil (1 tablespoon)

Organic brown sugar (1/2 cup)

Directions:

Combine sugars and cinnamon. Add oils and mix thoroughly.

Shelf Life: Store for up to a month in an air tight container.

Sweet Plum

Ingredients:

Plums (6)

Almond oil (1 teaspoon)

Organic brown sugar (1 cup)

Directions:

Puree the plums in a blender. Add almond oil and plums to sugar.

Shelf Life: Use immediately.

Neroli Lemon Grass

Ingredients:

Lemongrass oil (2 drops)

Neroli oil (2 drops)

Organic brown sugar (1/2 cup)

Directions:

Combine the ingredients in a bowl and mix thoroughly.

Shelf Life: Store for up to 6 months in an air tight container

Peach Meringue
Ingredients:

Peach (1 ripe)

Egg white (1)

Organic white sugar (1 cup)

Directions:

Purée the peach in a blender. Next, beat the egg white until stiff and then fold the peach purée into the egg white. Add the sugar and stir by hand.

Shelf life: Use immediately.

Vanilla Coconut
Ingredients:

Coconut oil (1 tablespoon)

Jojoba oil (2 tablespoons)

Vanilla fragrance oil (10 drops)

Coconut fragrance oil (10 drops)

Organic white sugar (1 cup)

Directions:

Combine the ingredients in a bowl and mix thoroughly.

Shelf Life: Store for up to 6 months in an air tight container

Field of Flowers
Ingredients:

Grapeseed oil (6-8 teaspoon)

Chamomile oil (2 drops)

Rose oil (2 drops)

Geranium oil (2 drops)

Jasmine oil (2 drops)

Organic white sugar (1 cup)

Directions:

Add oils to a mixing bowl of sugar. Mix thoroughly.

Shelf Life: Store for up to 1 week in an air tight container.

Lavender Apricot
Ingredients:

Organic white sugar (1/2 cup)

Plain yogurt (1/4 cup)

Mashed fresh apricots (1/8 cup)

Honey (1/8 cup)

Lavender essential oils (2 drops)

Directions:

Mix ingredients together in a large bowl.

Shelf Life: Store for 1 day in an air tight container.

Strawberry Daiquiri

Ingredients:

Very ripe fresh strawberries (1/2 cup)

Organic white sugar (1 cup)

Strawberry fragrance oil (2 drops)

Directions:

Puree strawberries and add fragrance oil and sugar.

Shelf Life: Store for a day in an air tight container.

Sweet Sage And Lemon

Ingredients:

Fresh sage (2 tablespoons)

Almond oil (4 tablespoons)

Lemon essential oil (2 drops)

Organic white sugar (1 cup)

Directions:

In a food processor, place sage or chop by hand until fine. Add the sugar and sage together in a mixing bowl and stir until sage is evenly distributed. Then add remaining ingredients and stir to mix.

Shelf life: Store and refrigerate for up to a week in an air tight container.

Almond Honey

Ingredients:

Crushed almonds (2 tablespoon)

Honey (1 tablespoon)

Organic brown sugar (1 cup)

Directions:

Place almonds in a food processor and chop until fine. In a mixing bowl, add almonds to remaining ingredients and stir to combine.

Shelf life: Store for up to a week in an air tight container

Lavender Lime
Ingredients:

Lime oil (3 drops)

Lavender oil (3 drops)

Organic white sugar (1 cup)

Directions:

Combine in a bowl and mix thoroughly.

Shelf Life: Store for up to 3 month in an air tight container.

Wheat Germ
Ingredients:

Cocoa butter (1/4 cup)

Organic wheat germ (1 tablespoon)

Apricot kernel oil (1 tablespoon)

Vitamin E oil (1 tablespoon)

Organic brown sugar (1/2)

Directions:

Use the double boiler method to melt the cocoa butter. Pour into a mixing bowl. Next, add remaining ingredients and stir to combine.

Shelf life: Store for up to 1 week in an air tight container.

Lemon Poppy
Ingredients:

Olive oil (1/2 cup)

Poppy seeds (1/2 cup)

Lemon essential oil (1/4 teaspoon)

Organic white sugar (1/2 cup)

Directions:

Thoroughly mix all of the ingredients together.

Shelf Life: Store for 1 month in an air tight container

Apple Honey
Ingredients:

Apple, cored, quartered (1)

Honey (2 tablespoon)

Teaspoon sage (1/2 tablespoon)

Organic white sugar (1 cup)

Directions:

Place the apple slices into a food processor and chop. Then, add honey, sage and sugar.

Shelf life: Use immediately.

Vanilla Rose
Ingredients:

Rosewater (2 tablespoon)

Vanilla fragrance oil (10 drops)

Rose fragrance oil (4 drops)

Organic white sugar (1 cup)

Directions:

Combine ingredients and mix well.

Shelf Life: Store for up to 1 month in an air tight container.

Grapeseed And Grapes
Ingredients:

Grapeseed oil (8 teaspoon)

White grapes (1/2 cup)

Organic white sugar (1 cup)

Directions:

Puree grapes in a blender. Next, add grapeseed oil, grapes to a mixing bowl of sugar. Mix thoroughly

Shelf Life: Store for up to 3 days in an air tight container

Jojoba Aloe Vera

Ingredients:

Jojoba oil (2 tablespoons)

Cocoa butter (2 tablespoon)

Vitamin E oil (1 tablespoon)

Aloe Vera gel (2 tablespoon)

Organic white sugar (1 cup)

Directions:

Combine in a bowl and mix thoroughly.

Shelf Life:

Store for up to 1 month in an air tight container.

Bananas Forrester

Ingredients:

Ripe banana (1)

Almond oil (1 tablespoon)

Organic white sugar (1/2 cup)

Organic brown sugar (1/2 cup)

Directions:

Puree banana in a blender. Then add sugars and blend till smooth. Pour into a bowl and mix in almond oil.

Shelf Life: Use immediately.

Godiva
<u>Ingredients:</u>

Godiva Chocolates (1 handful)

Organic white sugar (1/4 cup)

Peanut oil (2 tablespoon)

Fresh whole milk (2 tablespoon)

<u>Directions:</u>

Use the double boiler method to melt the chocolate. In a mixing bowl add the milk, sugar and peanut oil. Next, pour in chocolate and mix thoroughly.

Shelf Life: Store for up to 1 week in an air tight container

Honey Mint
<u>Ingredients:</u>

Mint (1 tablespoon)

Oil (1 tablespoon)

Honey (1 tablespoon)

Organic white sugar (1 cup)

<u>Directions:</u>

Finely chop the mint by hand or in a food processor. Add mint to sugars and other ingredients.

Shelf Life: Store for up to 1 month in an air tight container

Grapeseed and Avocado
Ingredients:

Grapeseed oil (8 teaspoon)

Avocado (1 ripe)

Organic white sugar (1 cup)

Directions:

Puree avocado in a blender. Then add grapeseed oil to a mixing bowl of sugar.

Mix thoroughly.

Shelf Life: Store for up to 3 days in an air tight container

Sweet Basil
Ingredients:

Basil oil (1 drop)

Fresh basil (2 tablespoons)

Organic white sugar (1 cup)

Directions:

Finely chop basil in food processor. Put all ingredients and mix well.

Shelf Life: Store for one day in an air tight container.

Citrus Sandalwood
Ingredients:

Safflower oil (10 teaspoon)

Orange blossom oil (5 drops)

Sandalwood oil (2 drops)

Organic brown sugar (1 cup)

<u>Directions</u>:

Mix ingredients together and pour into glass jars.

Shelf Life: Store for up to 3 months in an air tight container

SALT BODY SCRUBS

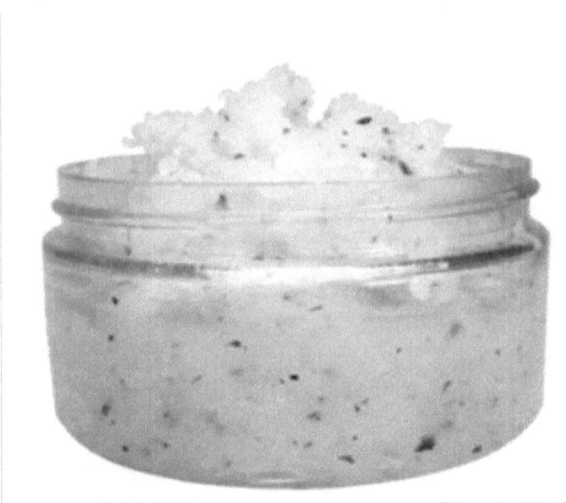

Salt scrubs enhance the circulation to the skin. They are coarser than sugar-based scrubs and have more exfoliating power.

People who have sensitive skin should not use salt scrubs. However, it is best to begin your exfoliating routine once a week.

Chamomile Jasmine
Ingredients:

Dried chamomile leaves (1 tablespoon)

Jasmine essential oil (1 tablespoon)

Crushed organic sea salt (1 cup)

Jojoba oil (3 tablespoon)

Directions:

Combine ingredients in mixing bowl and stir.

Shelf Life: Store for up to 1 week

Geranium

Ingredients:

Crushed organic sea salt (1/2 cup)

Geranium essential oil (4 drops)

Shea butter (2 tablespoons)

Apricot kernel oil (2 tablespoons)

Directions:

Use the double boiler method to melt Shea butter. Add to oils and sea salt

Shelf Life: Store for up to 6 months.

Artichoke

Ingredients:

Fresh artichoke hearts (1)

Canola oil (2 teaspoon)

Crushed organic sea salt (1 cup)

Fresh lemon juice (1 teaspoon)

Directions:

Mash cooked artichoke hearts in a glass bowl and mix with lemon and oil.

Stir well till smooth paste.

Shelf Life: Store for 1 week.

Mucho Mango

Ingredients:

Ripe mango (1)

Mango butter (2 tablespoon)

Crushed organic sea salt (1 cup)

Apricot kernel oil (2 tablespoons)

Directions:

Use the double boiler method to melt mango butter. Puree mango in a blender.

Mix all ingredients in a bowl and stir well.

Shelf Life: Store for 2 months.

Milk And Honey

Ingredients:

Milk or cream (1/4 cup)

Crushed organic sea salt (1 cup)

Honey (1/4 cup)

Directions:

Mix honey and milk (or cream) in an enamel pan or a small glass.

Warm until the honey melts. Remove from heat.

Shelf Life: Store for 1 week.

Cucumber Yogurt

Ingredients:

Cucumber (1 tablespoon)

Parsley (1 tablespoon)

Yogurt (1 tablespoon)

Crushed organic sea salt (1cup)

Directions:

Combine ingredients in mixing bowl and stir.

Almond Milk

Ingredients:

Almond oil (1/4 cup)

1 cup crushed organic sea salt (1 cup)

Almond milk (1/4 cup)

Directions:

Mix ingredients until well mixed.

Shelf Life: Store for 1 week.

Lavender Mint

Ingredients:

Dried lavender (2 tablespoons)

Mint (1 tablespoon)

Crushed organic sea salt (1cup)

Canola oil (4 tablespoons)

Directions:

Place mint on a cutting board and finely chop. Continue with salt, oil and dried lavender.

Shelf Life: Store for 3 months.

Raspberry
Ingredients:

Fresh raspberry (1/2 cup)

1 cup crushed organic sea salt (1 cup)

Sunflower oil (4 tablespoons)

Directions:

Combine ingredients in a food processor.

Shelf Life: Store in a glass jar for a week.

Summer Glow
Ingredients:

Crushed organic sea salt (1/2 cup)

Mango butter (2 tablespoons)

Shea butter (2 tablespoons)

Cocoa butter (2 tablespoons)

Fine silver glitter (1/2 tablespoons)

Directions:

Use the double boiler method to melt all the butters together.

Combine all ingredients in a bowl and use a hand mixer to mix well.

Shelf Life: Store for up to 2 months in an air tight container.

Apricot
Ingredients:

Crushed organic sea salt (1/2 cup)

Fresh apricot (1/2 cup)

Apricot fragrance oil (2 drops)

Directions:

Puree apricot in blender. Mix all ingredients in a bowl and stir well.

Shelf Life: Store for 1 week in an air tight container

Cinnamon And Spice
Ingredients:

Sunflower oil (4 tablespoon)

Crushed organic sea salt (1 cup)

Ground cinnamon (2 tablespoon)

Ground nutmeg (1 tablespoon)

Directions:

Combine ingredients in a bowl and mix thoroughly.

Shelf Life: Store for up to 2 months in an air tight container.

Eucalyptus
Ingredients:

Olive oil (4 tablespoon)

Crushed organic sea salt (1/2 cup)

Eucalyptus essential oil (2 drops)

Directions:

Combine ingredients in a bowl and mix thoroughly.

Shelf Life: Store for up to 6 months in an air tight container.

Milk And Herbs
Ingredients:

Olive oil (4 tablespoon)

Crushed organic sea salt (1/2cup)

Powdered goats milk (2 tablespoon)

Dried thyme (1 tablespoon)

Dried rosemary (1 tablespoon)

Directions:

Combine ingredients in a bowl and mix thoroughly.

Shelf Life: Store for 2 weeks in an air tight container.

Oats And Honey

Ingredients:

Powdered oats (1/4 cup)

Crushed organic sea salt (1/2 cup)

Honey (1/4 cup)

Sweet almond (2 tablespoons)

Directions:

Mix powdered oats and salt. Add the honey and then the oil.

Mix until fully combined.

Shelf Life: Store for 2 months in an air tight container.

Watermelon Splash

Ingredients:

Crushed organic sea salt (1/2 cup)

Fresh watermelon (1/2 cup)

Directions:

Combine ingredients in a bowl and mix well.

Shelf Life: Store for up to 1 week in an air tight container.

Pomegranate

Ingredients:

Apricot kernel oil (4 tablespoon)

Crushed organic sea salt (1 cup)

Pomegranate juice (2 tablespoon)

Pomegranate fragrance oil (3 drop)

Directions:

Combine ingredients in a bowl and mix well.

Shelf Life: Store for up to 2 weeks in an air tight container.

Fruit And Nut
Ingredients:

Crushed almonds (1/2 cup)

Crushed organic sea salt (1/2 cup)

Raisons (2 tablespoons)

Dried cranberries (2)

Almond oil (2 tablespoon)

Directions:

Combine ingredients in a bowl and mix thoroughly.

Shelf Life: Store for 2 months in an air tight container.

Tangerine Mint
 Ingredients:

Olive oil (4 tablespoon)

Cup crushed organic sea salt (1/2cup)

Tangerine fragrance oil (2 drops)

Spearmint essential oil (2 drops)

Directions:

Combine all ingredients and mix well.

Shelf Life: Store for up to 6 months in an air tight container.

Ginger Lime
Ingredients:

Crushed organic sea salt (1 cup)

Ground ginger (1 teaspoon)

Fresh lime juice (1 teaspoon)

Macadamia nut oil (4 tablespoon)

Directions:

Combine all ingredients and mix well.

Shelf Life: Store for up to 2 weeks in an air tight container.

Very Berry
Ingredients:

Strawberry fragrance oil (2 drops)

Crushed organic sea salt (1 cup)

Raspberry fragrance oil (2 drops)

Sweet almond oil (2 tablespoon)

Vitamin E oil (2 tablespoon)

Directions:

Combine all the ingredients in a bowl and stir well.

Shelf Life: Store for up to 3 months in a glass jar.

Vanilla Milk
Ingredients:

Vanilla extract (2 tablespoon)

Crushed organic sea salt (1 cup)

Milk (4 tablespoons)

Powdered goat's milk (2 tablespoon)

Directions:

Mix all the ingredients in a glass bowl.

Shelf Life: Store for up to 1 week in a glass jar.

Hazel Nut
Ingredients:

Crushed organic sea salt (1/2 cup)

Hazel nut oil (2 tablespoon)

Crushed hazel nuts (1/4)

Directions:

Mix all ingredients.

Shelf Life: Store for a week in an air tight container.

Tomato Carrot
Ingredients:

Crushed organic sea salt (1/2 cup)

Ripe tomato (1)

Carrot juice (1/4)

Directions:

Puree carrot juice and tomato. Add salt and beat with a hand mixer.

Shelf Life: Store for up to 1 week in an air tight container.

Citrus Blend

Ingredients:

Mango butter (2 tablespoon)

Crushed organic sea salt (1 cup)

Orange essential oil (2 drops)

Lemon essential oil (2 drops)

Grapefruit essential oil (2 drops)

Almond oil (2 tablespoon)

Directions:

Use a double boiler to melt mango butter and add to the other ingredients.

Shelf Life: Store for up to 6 months in an air tight container.

Tangerine

Ingredients:

Tangerine essential oil (2 drop)

Crushed organic sea salt (1 cup)

Dried orange peel powder (4 tablespoons)

Apricot kernel (2 tablespoons)

Directions:

Mix all the ingredients and stir well.

Shelf Life: Store for up to 3 months in a glass jar.

Egyptian Nights
Ingredients:

Crushed organic sea salt (1/2 cup)

Egyptian musk fragrance oil (3 drops)

Epsom salt (1/4 cup)

Directions:

Combine all ingredients and mix well

Shelf Life: Store for up to 6 months in an air tight container.

Frankincense And Sandalwood
Ingredients:

Frankincense essential oil (2 drops)

Crushed organic sea salt (1 cup)

Sandalwood essential oil (2 drops)

Vegetable oil (2 tablespoon)

Directions:

Mix all ingredients in a bowl and stir well.

Shelf Life: Store for up to 3 months in a glass jar.

Rosemary Soy Milk

Ingredients:

Soy milk (2 tablespoon)

Crushed organic sea salt (1 cup)

Dried rosemary (4 tablespoons)

Canola oil (4 tablespoons)

Directions:

Mix all ingredients in a glass bowl.

Shelf Life: Store for up to 1 week in a glass jar.

Pink Champagne

Ingredients:

French pink champagne (2 tablespoon)

Crushed organic sea salt (1 cup)

Epsom salt (2 tablespoon)

Directions:

Mix all ingredients in a glass bowl.

Shelf Life: Store for up to 2 weeks in a glass jar.

Banana Berry

Ingredients:

Ripe banana (1)

Strawberry fragrance oil (3 drops)

Crushed organic sea salt (1/2 cup)

Fresh strawberries (1/4)

Directions:

Combine all ingredients and mix with a hand mixer.

Shelf Life: Store for 2 days in an air tight container

Buttermilk

Ingredients:

Crushed organic sea salt (1/2 cup)

Lemon tea tree essential oil (1 teaspoon)

Buttermilk (2 teaspoon)

Yogurt (2 teaspoons)

Directions:

Mix all ingredients in a mixing bowl.

Shelf Life: Store for a week in an air tight container.

Autumn Harvest
Ingredients:

Peach fragrance oil (3 drops)

Bergamot Essential Oil (3 drops)

Vanilla Essential Oil (3 drops)

Range fragrance oil (3 drops)

Crushed organic sea salt (1/2 cup)

Directions:

Combine all ingredients and mix.

Shelf Life: Store for up to 6 months in an air tight container.

Rose Bouquet
Ingredients:

Pink Rose Petal Powder (2 tablespoon)

Crushed organic sea salt (1 cup)

Rose fragrance oil (3 drops)

Rosewater Powder (1 tablespoon)

Directions:

Combine all ingredients in a mixing bowl.

Shelf Life: Store for 2 months.

Herb Butter

Ingredients:

Dried mint (2 teaspoon)

Dried sage (2 teaspoon)

Dried rosemary (2 teaspoon)

Cocoa butter (6 ounces)

Crushed organic sea salt (1 cup)

Directions:

Combine all ingredients in a mixing bowl.

Shelf Life: Store for 6 months.

Cucumber Lemon

Ingredients:

Crushed organic sea salt (1/2 cup)

Ripe cucumber (1)

Fresh squeezed lemon juice (2 tablespoon)

Yogurt (2 tablespoon)

Lemon essential oil (2 drops)

Directions:

Chop cucumber into small pieces, add yogurt and lemon then blend to make a paste.

Next, remove from food processor and add salt. Mix thoroughly.

Shelf Life: Store for a week in an air tight container.

Rosemary Peppermint
Ingredients:

Dried rosemary (2 tablespoon)

Crushed organic sea salt (1 cup)

Peppermint fragrance oil (3 drops)

Directions:

Combine all ingredients in a mixing bowl.

Shelf Life: Store for 6 months.

Jasmine and Violet
Ingredients:

Jasmine essential Oil (3 drops)

Violet essential Oil (3 drops)

Crushed organic sea salt (1/2 cup)

Directions:

Combine ingredients in a bowl and mix.

Shelf Life: Store in an air tight container for 6 months.

Hot Buttered Corn
Ingredients:

Crushed organic sea salt (1/2 cup)

Butter (1 teaspoon)

Canola oil (1 teaspoon)

Corn meal (11/4 cup)

Water (11/4 cup)

Directions:

Microwave the cornmeal and water for 1 minute on high temperature.

Combine the remaining ingredients in a mixing bowl.

Leave to cool till room temperature.

Shelf Life: Store in an air tight container for a month.

Autumn Harvest
Ingredients:

Peach fragrance oil (3 drops)

Bergamot Essential Oil (3 drops)

Vanilla Essential Oil (7drops)

Orange fragrance oil (3 drops)

Crushed organic sea salt (1/2 cup)

Directions:

Combine ingredients in a bowl and mix.

Shelf Life: Store for up to 6 months in an air tight container.

Sweet And Salty
Ingredients:

Crushed organic sea salt (1/2 cup)

Organic white sugar (1/2 cup)

Directions:

Combine all ingredients and beat.

Shelf Life: Store for up to 1 week in an air tight container.

Rose Rosemary

Ingredients:

Rose essential oil (3 drops)

Crushed organic sea salt (1/2 cup)

Dried rosemary (2 tablespoon)

Directions:

Combine ingredients and beat with a hand mixer.

Shelf Life: Store in an air tight container for a week.

Apple Pear

Ingredients:

Crushed organic sea salt (1/2 cup)

Small fresh green apple (1)

Small pear (1)

Fresh lemon (2 teaspoons)

Apple fragrance oil (2 drops)

Pear fragrance oil (2 drops)

Directions:

Puree fruit with lemon juice in a blender. Then, combine all ingredients and mix thoroughly.

Shelf Life: Store for a day in an air tight container.

Sweet Potato
Ingredients:

Crushed organic sea salt (1/2 cup)

Cooked sweet potato (1/2 cup)

Ground cinnamon (1 teaspoon)

Directions:

Combine ingredients and beat with a hand mixer.

Shelf Life: Store in an air tight container for to 2 weeks.

Cranberry Almond
Ingredients:

Crushed almonds (1/2 cup)

Crushed organic sea salt (1/2 cup)

Cranberries (2)

Almond oil (2 tablespoon)

Directions:

Combine ingredients in a bowl and mix well.

Shelf Life: Store in an air tight container for 2 months.

Beer And Mayonnaise
<u>Ingredients:</u>

Beer (1/2 cup)

Crushed organic sea salt (1/2 cup)

Mayonnaise (2 tablespoon)

<u>Directions:</u>

Combine all ingredients and beat with a hand mixer.

Shelf Life: Store in an air tight container for 2 weeks.

Pineapple Passion
<u>Ingredients:</u>

Pineapple fragrance oil (3 drops)

Passion fruit fragrance oil (3 drops)

Crushed organic sea salt (1/2 cup)

Fresh pineapple (1/2 cup)

<u>Directions:</u>

Puree fruits in the blender. Mix all ingredients in a bowl and beat with a hand mixer.

Shelf Life: Store in an air tight container for a week.

Egg Protein
<u>Ingredients:</u>

Crushed organic sea salt (1/2 cup)

Large egg (1)

Protein powder (2 tablespoon)

Directions:

Combine ingredients and beat with a hand mixer.

Shelf Life: Store in an air tight container for 2 months.

Strawberry Kiwi

Ingredients:

Strawberry fragrance (3 drops)

Crushed organic sea salt (1/2 cup)

Fresh strawberries (1/4 cup)

Ripe kiwi (1)

Directions:

Combine ingredients and beat with a hand mixer.

Shelf Life: Store for up to 1 week in an air tight container.

OATMEAL BODY SCRUBS

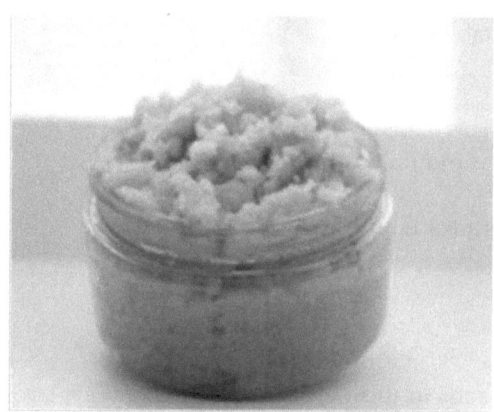

Oats contain grainy substances which have been proven to be very good for facial scrubs. Oats also absorb and remove surface dirt and skin impurities.

Using scrubs made with this wonderful ingredient will help in treating several skin conditions. It works well for dry and itchy skin and is just right for sensitive skin.

Scrubs used with oatmeal will leave your skin soft, silky smooth and hydrated.

Before applying any oatmeal scrub, it is advisable to wash your face with lukewarm water. The scrub can also be used immediately after a shower. This opens up the pores and prepares the skin for improved result.

Grapefruit & Oatmeal Scrub

The use of citrus with oatmeal is a wonderful combination that helps in stimulating, toning and exfoliating the skin.

<u>Ingredients</u>

Fresh Grapefruit (1)

63

Oatmeal (2 tablespoons)

Directions:

Squeeze juice and pulp out of grapefruit.

Mix with oatmeal till it forms a smooth paste.

Baking Soda & Oatmeal Scrub

The baking soda in this oatmeal scrub serves as a booster. It will soothe your skin in a pleasantly surprising way.

Ingredients

Oatmeal (2 heaping tablespoons)

Baking soda (1 teaspoon)

Directions:

Mix ingredients and add sufficient water to make a sticky paste.

Scrub your face in circular motions, massaging it gently to your skin. Rinse off with lukewarm water.

Oatmeal Sunset Glow

The honey included in this scrub is a natural humectant. It absorbs moisture and keeps it under your skin –just where it ought to be. The apple cider vinegar restores your skin's natural acidity. Vinegar is ideal for both dry and oily complexions as it will keep it softy and fresh.

Ingredients

Oatmeal (8 tablespoons)

Apple cider Vinegar (1 tablespoon)

Dark organic Honey (1 tablespoon)

Finely ground Almonds (2 teaspoon)

Direction:

Put honey in a metal bowl or small glass then warm it in microwave till it becomes runny.

Mix all ingredients until you have a smooth paste

Oatmeal And More

The rich ingredients below is a peek of what to expect –it soothes, exfoliates, cleanse, moisturizes and more!

Ingredients:

Medium Cucumber (1/4 peeled)

Plain unflavored Yogurt (2 tablespoons)

Oatmeal (2 tablespoons)

Jojoba oil　(1 teaspoon)

Sweet Almond oil (1 teaspoon)

Direction:

Slice cucumber and whizz in food processor till it's liquefied.

Add remaining ingredients and mix to make a smooth paste.

Almonds, Avocado & Oatmeal Scrub

Use this avocado based scrub and see how smooth, soft, hydrated and nourished your skin will feel.

Ingredients:

Oatmeal (1 cup)

Coarsely ground Almonds (1 tablespoon)

Peeled ripe Avocado (1)

Direction:

Mix the grounded almonds and oatmeal. Next, mash the peeled avocado to a pulp.

Dip avocado pulp in the almond, oatmeal mix.

Rub and massage on your face very gently, then rinse off.

Cheesy& Juicy Oatmeal Scrub
Cream cheese contains lactic acid that tones and cleanses the skin

Ingredients:

Oatmeal (2 tablespoons)

Cream cheese (1 tablespoon)

Fresh Lemon juice (1 teaspoon)

Direction:

Mix all ingredients until it forms a creamy paste.

Oatmeal &Peels Scrub
A rejuvenating scrub for those who want to smell fresh all day long

Ingredients:

Dried Orange peels (1 cup)

Oatmeal (1 cup)

Finely ground Almonds (2 tablespoon)

Sweet Orange essential oil (1 teaspoon)

Direction:

Put ingredients in a food processor and mix thoroughly. Take a little of this mix in your hand, add some warm water and make a paste. Rub and massage onto your skin.

Cornstarch, Oatmeal And More
A soothing and relaxing body scrub

Ingredients:

Almonds (1/4 cup)

Oatmeal (4 tablespoons)

Cornstarch (1 tablespoon)

Lavender essential oil (2 teaspoons)

Crushed dried Chamomile flowers (1 tablespoon)

Directions:

Place all ingredients in a food processor.

Blend and mash them well.

Take half a tablespoon of this mix in your hand. Add water to make a paste

Cranberries, Coconut Super Oatmeal Scrub
Cranberries have everything your skin needs. Their inclusion in this recipe will help to exfoliate and clean your pores.

The coconut oil is not as greasy as other moisturizers. It is also very effective.

Ingredients

Cranberries (1/2 cup)

Oatmeal (4 tablespoons)

Coconut oil (2 tablespoons)

Sweet Almond oil (1 tablespoon)

Extra virgin Olive oil (1 tablespoon)

Brown Sugar (2 tablespoons)

Directions

Put ingredients in a food processor and mash and blend well.

www.ingramcontent.com/pod-product-compliance
Lightning Source LLC
Chambersburg PA
CBHW022345290526
45786CB00014B/2505